Farès Azaiez

Spontaneous coronary artery dissection

Farès Azaiez

Spontaneous coronary artery dissection

Treatment and long-term prognosis

ScienciaScripts

Imprint
Any brand names and product names mentioned in this book are subject to trademark, brand or patent protection and are trademarks or registered trademarks of their respective holders. The use of brand names, product names, common names, trade names, product descriptions etc. even without a particular marking in this work is in no way to be construed to mean that such names may be regarded as unrestricted in respect of trademark and brand protection legislation and could thus be used by anyone.

Cover image: www.ingimage.com

This book is a translation from the original published under ISBN 978-620-6-72484-1.

Publisher:
Sciencia Scripts
is a trademark of
Dodo Books Indian Ocean Ltd. and OmniScriptum S.R.L publishing group

120 High Road, East Finchley, London, N2 9ED, United Kingdom
Str. Armeneasca 28/1, office 1, Chisinau MD-2012, Republic of Moldova, Europe
Printed at: see last page
ISBN: 978-620-8-18604-3

Table of contents

LIST OF ABBREVIATIONS

- **ARB II**: angiotensin II receptor antagonist
- **STROKE :** Cerebrovascular accident
- **CD:** right coronary
- **Cx:** circumflex
- **FMD:** fibromuscular dysplasia
- **Dg**: diagonal
- **DSAC:** spontaneous dissection of the coronary arteries
- **ECG:** electrocardiogram
- **TTE:** trans-thoracic echocardiography
- **LVEF**: left ventricular ejection fraction
- **CVRF:** cardiovascular risk factor
- **IMH:** intramural haematoma
- **HTA:** high blood pressure
- **PCI:** percutaneous coronary intervention
- **MI:** myocardial infarction
- **ACE** inhibitor: enzyme conversion inhibitor
- **AIV:** anterior interventricular
- **Mg:** marginal
- **NSTEMI:** non-ST-segment elevation myocardial infarction
- **OCT**: optical coherence tomography
- **CABG:** coronary artery bypass grafting
- **ACS:** acute coronary syndrome
- **STEMI:** myocardial infarction with persistent ST-segment elevation
- **TCG:** left common trunk

INTRODUCTION

Spontaneous coronary artery dissection (SCAD) is defined as dissection of an epicardial artery that is neither iatrogenic nor post-traumatic and not associated with atherosclerosis. The predominant mechanism of myocardial injury following SCAD is coronary obstruction caused by intramural haematoma (IMH) formation or intimal tear rather than intraluminal thrombus or atherosclerotic plaque rupture.

Since Pretty's first autopsy description of CASD in 1931 (1) in a 42-year-old woman who died following incoercible vomiting, our understanding of the disease has evolved enormously over the last eight decades, and particularly over the last five years.

Indeed, advances in our analysis of the epidemiology of CASD, the availability of endocoronary imaging techniques (2), the development of angiographic classification specific to CASD (3) and the watchful eye of interventional cardiologists suggest that CASD is much more common than previously thought, particularly in young women.

CASD therefore poses the problem of a diagnosis that is often confusing due to a different terrain, and therefore requires a different treatment and prognosis from atherosclerotic disease.

Our study was essentially based on the recent 2018 European (4) and American (5) consensus with the following objectives:

- Describe the demographic, clinical, angiographic and therapeutic characteristics of patients with CADS.
- Assess the immediate and long-term prognosis of these patients.

METHODS

I - TYPE OF STUDY

This was a single-centre prospective observational study conducted in the cardiology department of Mongi Slim La Marsa Hospital over a two-year period from August 2018 to August 2020.

II - STUDY POPULATION

Inclusion criteria :

The DSAC refers to the acute development of a false lumen in the wall of the coronary artery, which can compromise coronary flow by external compression of the true lumen; for this reason, only dissections discovered in the aftermath of acute coronary syndromes (ACS) have been included.

The angiographic appearance corresponded to one of the three types of the 2014 Saw et al. (3) classification or to type 4 completing this classification established in 2017 by Al-Hussaini and Adlam in 2017 (6).

Non-inclusion criteria :

Iatrogenic dissections, post-traumatic dissections or dissections resulting from primary aortic dissection, penetrating ulcers or ruptured atherosclerotic plaques were not included.

III - METHODOLOGY :

III-1-Data collection

CASD cases were prospectively collected since July 2018 from patients undergoing coronary angiography at the catheterization suite of Mongi Slim La Marsa Hospital.

The angiographic examinations were carried out and reviewed by the same operator.

We kept the patients' medical records after obtaining their consent for inclusion.

Prospective follow-up of all patients was recorded during subsequent consultations by the attending physicians or, failing that, by telephone contact.

- *Case history :*

Socio-demographic data, medical history and cardiovascular risk factors (CVRFs) were recorded.

In addition, the circumstances of onset, associated conditions and favouring factors described in the literature were investigated: pregnancy, fibromuscular dysplasia, connective tissue anomalies, systemic diseases and possible physical or emotional stress.

- Cardiovascular and general somatic examinations :

All patients underwent a cardiovascular examination with a 17-lead electrocardiogram (ECG).

Hospital complications of ACS, in particular haemodynamic and rhythmic complications, were identified.

- *Biology :*

Peak levels of markers of myocardial necrosis, in particular those of ultra-sensitive troponins, were recorded in order to stratify the risk of ACS without persistent ST-segment shift.

In addition, all patients had their blood count, renal function and ionogram, fasting blood sugar and lipid levels tested.

- *Transthoracic echocardiography :*

All patients underwent transthoracic echocardiography (TTE) to assess left ventricular ejection fraction (LVEF), segmental kinetics and possible complications of myocardial infarction (MI).

- *Coronary angiography :*

➔ *DSAC angiographic classification*

The National Heart, Lung, and Blood Institute (NHLBI) classification (7) was proposed before the era of stents to classify angioplasty-related dissections.

The classification specific to CASDs is that of Saw et al. (3) in three types (Figure 1) to which type 4 was added by Al-Hussaini and Adlam in 2017 (6).

TYPE 1: This is the pathognomonic angiographic appearance of SCAD with contrast of the arterial wall with visualisation of several lumens and radiolucent intimal flap.

TYPE 2: (Diffuse stenosis of varying severity): the angiographic appearance is not obvious and is often misdiagnosed. This dissection (typically > 20 mm) often involves the middle to distal segments of the coronary and may be so extensive that it reaches the distal end. There is an abrupt (often subtle) change in arterial calibre, with demarcation from normal diameter to diffuse narrowing.

TYPE 3: This appearance is the most difficult to differentiate from atherosclerosis and the most likely to be misdiagnosed, often requiring endocoronary imaging to confirm the diagnosis. The angiographic features that favour CASD are: (a) absence of atherosclerotic involvement in other arteries, (b) long lesions (11-20 mm), (c) cloudy stenosis and (d) linear stenosis.

TYPE 4: Occlusion (usually distal) of the vessel. An embolic cause must be ruled out in this presentation.

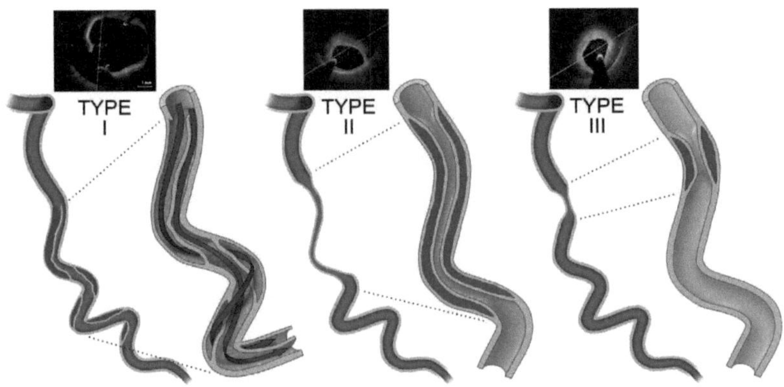

Figure 1: The first three types of spontaneous coronary dissection (8)

➔ Other lesion characteristics

We looked for coronary tortuosities and any intramyocardial tracts.

The definition used for coronary tortuosities is that of Eleid et al (9) proposed in 2014. Tortuosity was defined by the presence of at least three consecutive curvatures of 90° to 180° measured at end-diastole in a major epicardial coronary artery ≥ 2 mm in diameter (Figure 2).

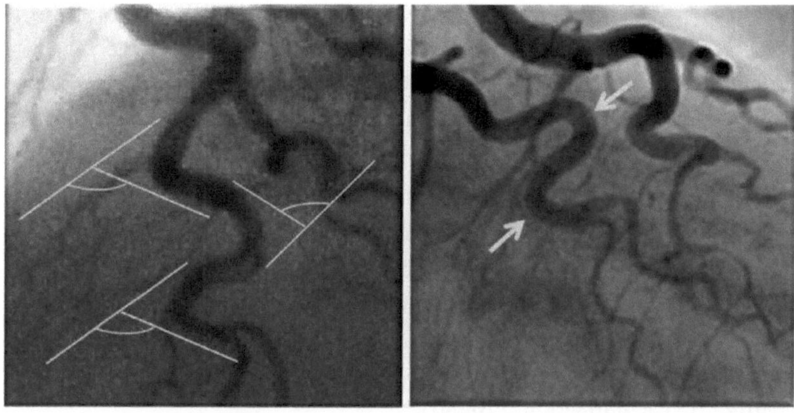

Figure 2: Definition of coronary tortuosity

- Therapeutic strategies :

Treatments initially administered before coronary angiography and after the diagnosis of CAD were recorded.

Patients either received conservative treatment alone or a coronary reperfusion strategy.

III-2- Definitions

➢ **Acute coronary syndrome:** The term ACS referred to any group of clinical symptoms consistent with acute myocardial ischaemia. It has included unstable angina, non persistent ST elevation myocardial infarction (NSTEMI) and ST elevation myocardial infarction (STEMI).

➢ **Major Adverse Cardiac and Cerebrovascular Events (MACCE)** (10)**:** defined as the occurrence of death from any cause, non-fatal MI, repeated revascularisation of the target vessel or stroke.

III-3- Judging criteria

The primary outcome was the occurrence of MACCE during the follow-up period.

III-4- Statistical methodology

We calculated simple frequencies and relative frequencies for the qualitative variables.

We calculated means, medians and standard deviations and determined the range (extreme values = minimum and maximum) for the quantitative variables.

IV. Bibliographical research

The search engines used in our study were PubMed (Medline) and ScienceDirect.

The keywords used in French were : Spontaneous coronary artery dissection, Myocardial revascularisation, Prognosis.

The key words used in English were: Spontaneous coronary artery dissection, myocardial revascularisation, Outcome.

V. Ethical considerations

We declare that we have had no conflicts of interest and that we have respected medical confidentiality for all cases that have been treated in our department.

VI. Writing the dissertation

We have followed the IMRAD format for scientific writing.

RESULTS

During the period under review, **13 cases of CASD** were diagnosed.

I - IMPACT

During the study period,1,473 coronary angiographies were performed, including 500 in the context of ACS.

The incidence of CASD was 0.9% of all coronary angiographies and 2.6% of coronary angiographies performed for ACS.

II - GENERAL CHARACTERISTICS OF THE POPULATION

II- 1 - Age

The mean age was 56 years, with a standard deviation of 11 years and extremes ranging from 35 to 72 years. Patients in their fifties were the most represented category.

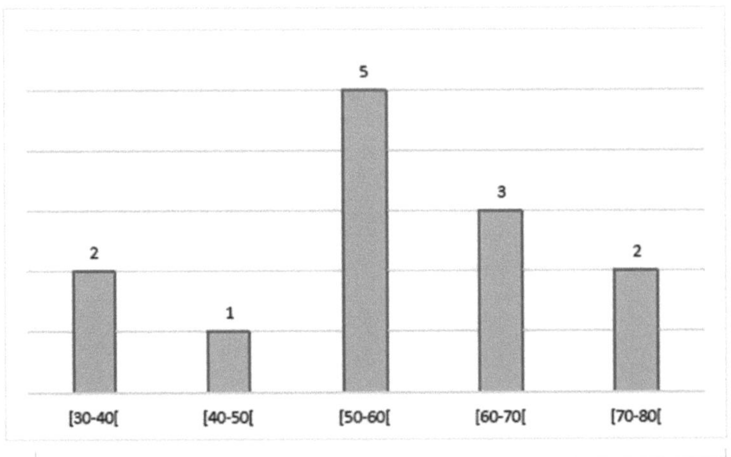

Figure 3: Breakdown of patients by age group.

II- 2 - Type

In our series, women predominated, with a sex ratio of 0.2.

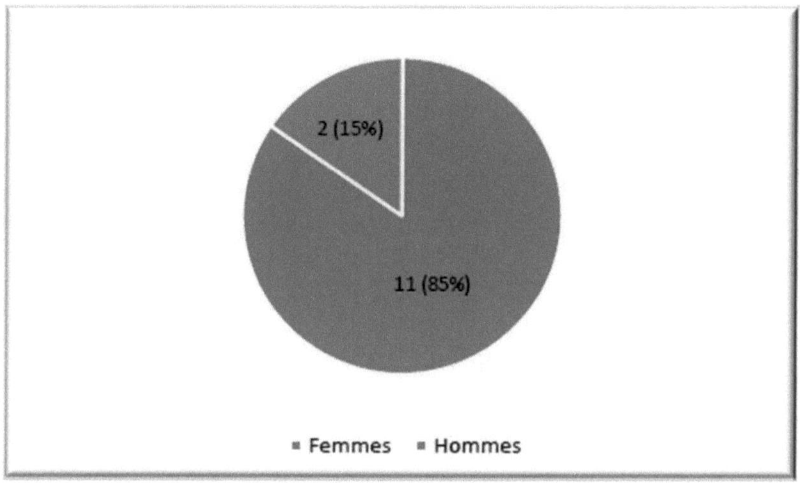

Figure 4: Breakdown of patients by gender.

II- 3- Cardiovascular risk factors

The majority of patients (N=6, 46%) had no FRCV.

Five patients had a single CVRF, one patient had two CVRFs and one patient had three CVRFs (Figure 5). Hypertension was the most common CVRF (5 patients, 38%) (Figure 6).

The average number of FRCVs per patient was 0.8.

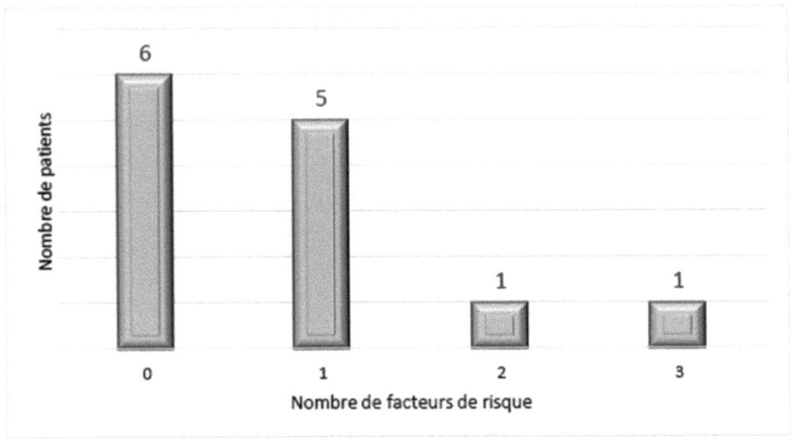

Figure 5: Association of cardiovascular risk factors.

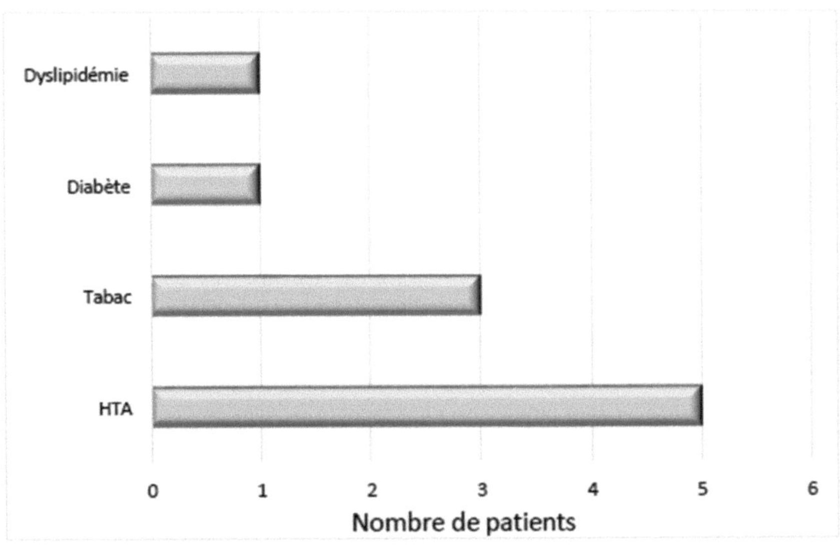

Figure 6: Prevalence of cardiovascular risk factors.

II- 4- Contributing factors and associated conditions

No cases of DSAC were related to pregnancy.

Intense physical stress and a hypertensive crisis were the causes in two patients each (Table I).

It should be noted that two patients had hypothyroidism under treatment.

Table I: Contributing factors and associated conditions

Associated conditions	Number of patients
Physical stress	2
Emotional stress	0
Hypertensive flare-up	2
Recreational drugs	0
Pregnancy	0
Systemic inflammatory disease	0
Fibromuscular dysplasia	0
Connective tissue disease	0
Depression	1
Migraine	1
Hypothyroidism	2

II- 5- Clinical and echocardiographic presentations

The predominant clinical presentation was NSTEMI in eight patients (61%). Of these, only one was at very high risk due to diffuse ST-segment undershoot with concomitant AVR overshoot.

Five patients (39%) had a STEMI, three of whom were progressive and two of whom were seen on day 2. Of the three patients with an active STEMI, two underwent thrombolysis with failure and subsequently underwent coronary angiography, while only one underwent coronary angiography immediately (Figure 7).

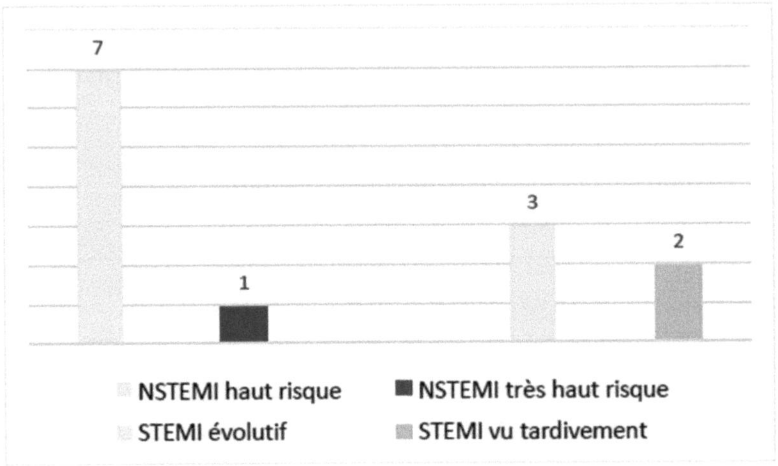

Figure 7: Clinical presentations on admission

The majority of patients (N=11, 85%) had normal segmental kinetics on TTE.

One patient had apical akinesia with a left intraventricular thrombus and another patient had segmental hypokinesia.

III - ANGIOGRAPHIC CHARACTERISTICS OF LESIONS

III - 1- Location of lesions

DSAC lesions mainly involved the anterior interventricular (AIV)-diagonal (Dg) axis (7 patients, 54%) followed by the circumflex (Cx)-marginal (Mg) and then the right coronary (RC) (Figure 8).

The left common trunk was not affected in our series.

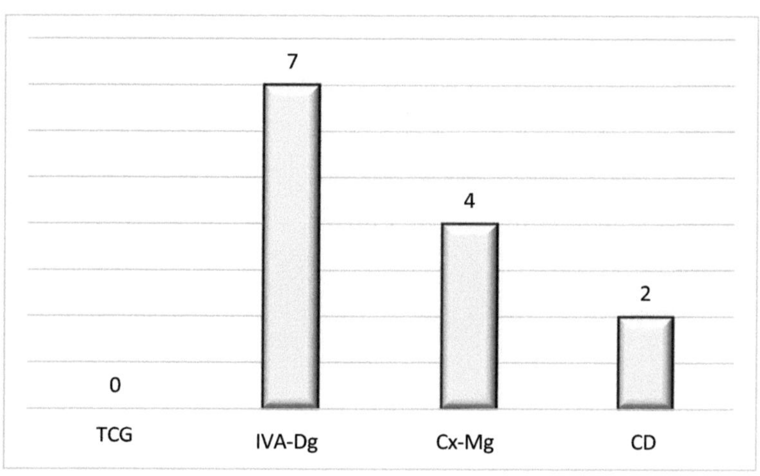

Figure 8: Location of spontaneous coronary artery dissection lesions

III - 2 - Characteristics of lesions

The majority of patients had a type 2 DSAC (46%) with a length >20 mm (62%) (Table II).

Severe tortuosity was associated with 5 patients (38%).

Table II: Main lesion characteristics

Features	Number of patients (%)
Angiographic type *	
• Type 1	5 (38)
• Type 2	6 (46)
• Type 3	1 (8)
• Type 4	1 (8)
Length (mm)	
• <10	3 (23)
• 10-20	2 (15)
• >20	8 (62)
Thrombus	2 (15)
Severe tortuosity	5 (38)
Intramyocardial pathway	0 (0)

* : according to the classification of Saw et al.

III- 3- Angiographic images

The different angiographic presentations of the 13 patients are shown in Figures 9 to 21.

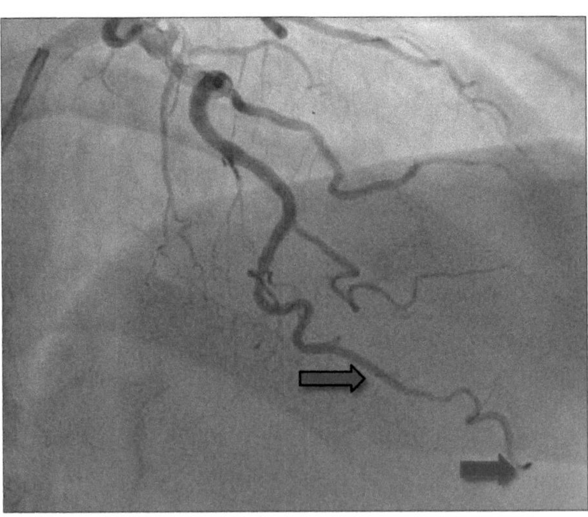

- Figure 9: 71-year-old woman, hypertensive dyslipidaemic, electrical syndrome of the VIA. **Type 2 dissection of the distal VIA.**

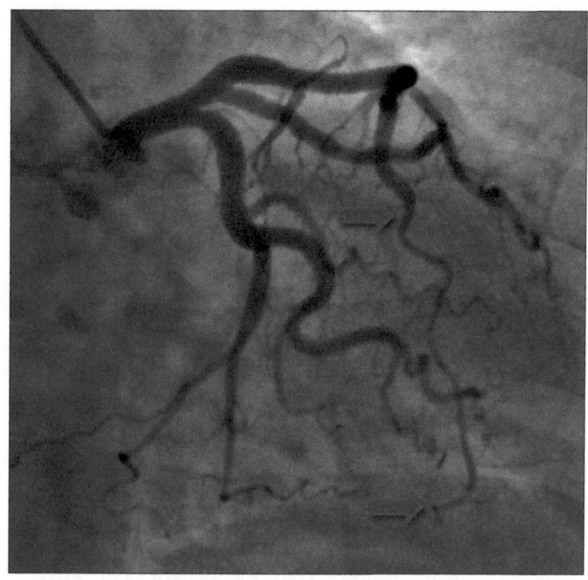

Figure 10: 63-year-old woman, hypertensive smoker, apicolateral subepicardial ischaemia. **Type 2 dissection of the distal LAI.**

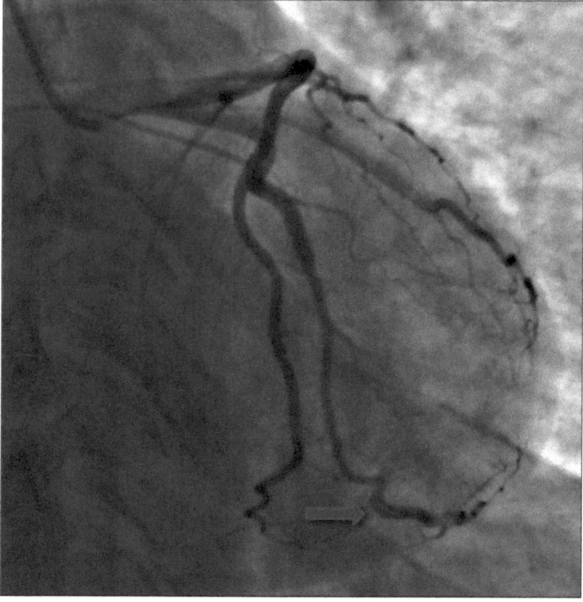

Figure 11: 48-year-old woman, inferior subepicardial ischaemia. **Type 1 dissection of the distal Mg.**

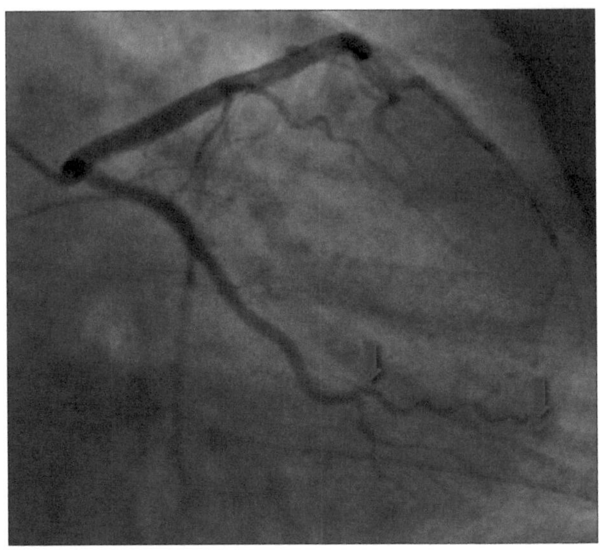

Figure 12: 56-year-old woman, basal MI. **Type 2 dissection of the distal Mg** confirmed on MRI (transmural ischaemic contrast ofthe medioventricular lateral wall).

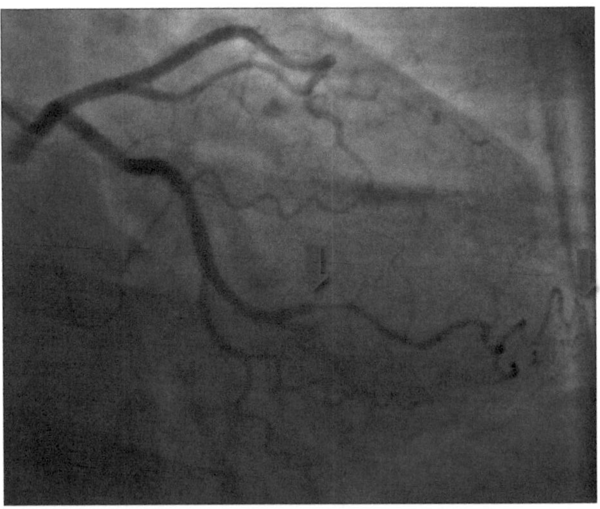

Figure 13: 50-year-old woman, smoker, hypertensive, NSTEMI with normal ECG. **Type 2 dissection of the distal Mg**.

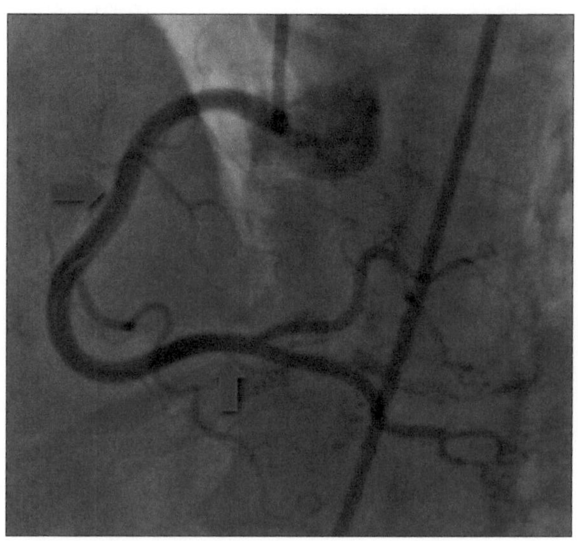

Figure 14: 60-year-old woman, hypertensive dyslipidaemic diabetic, NSTEMI with normal ECG. **Type 1 dissection of CD II-III.**

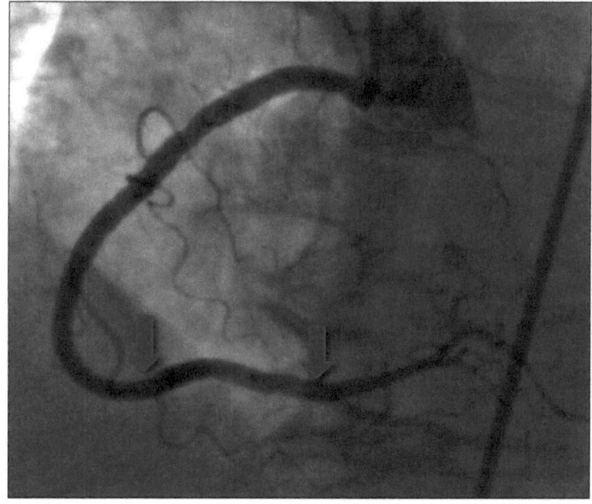

Figure 15: 67-year-old woman, inferobasal MI. **Type 1 dissection of CD III.**

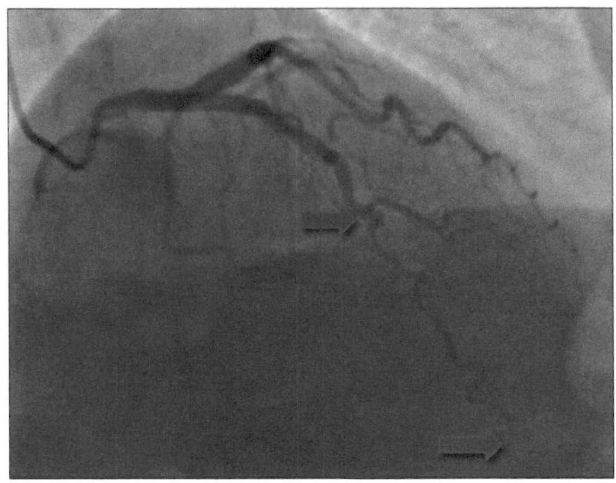

Figure 16: 72-year-old woman, NSTEMI with normal ECG. **Type 2 dissection of IVA III**.

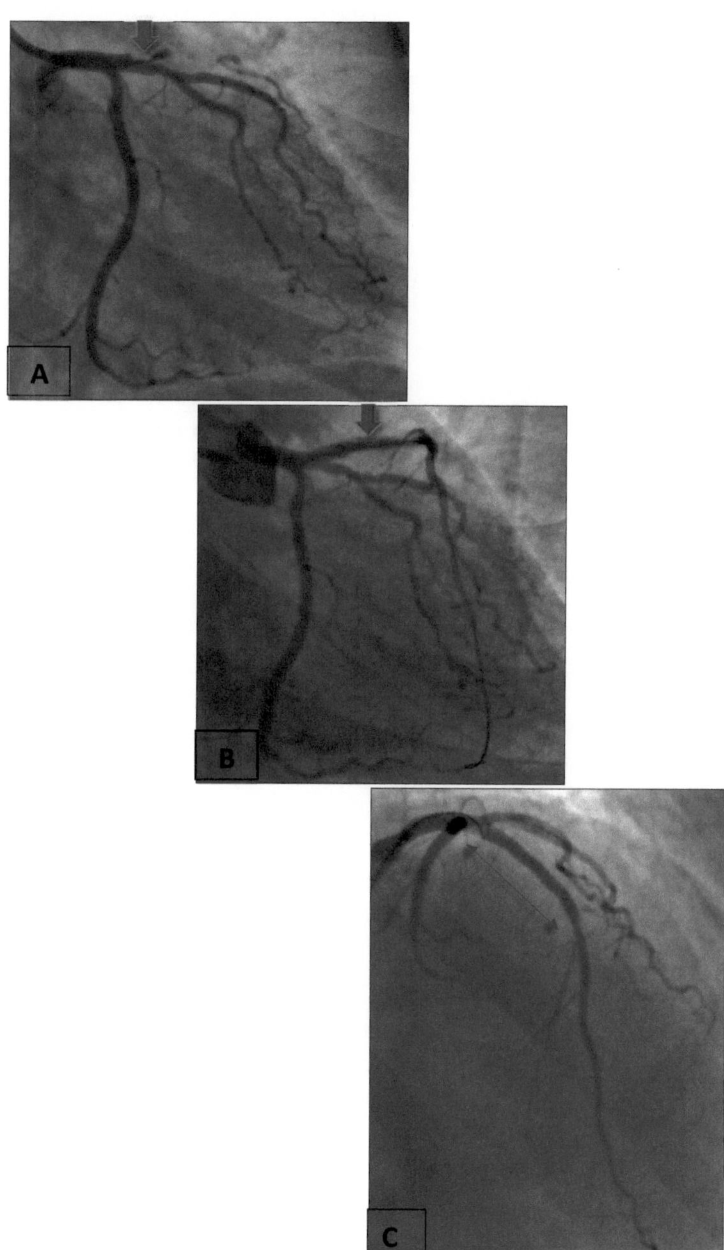

Figure 17: 59-year-old woman, previous MI. **Type 4 dissection of IVA I** (A). Intimal flap after thromboaspiration (B). Final result after angioplasty with a long active stent (C).

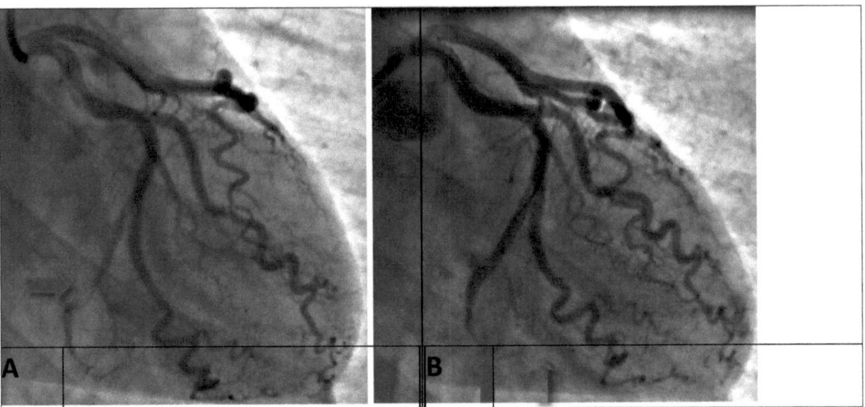

Figure 18: 57-year-old woman, smoker, apicolateral MI. **Type 1 dissection of the distal Cx** (A). Final result after stent angioplasty with migration of the haematoma distally and occlusion of the artery (B).

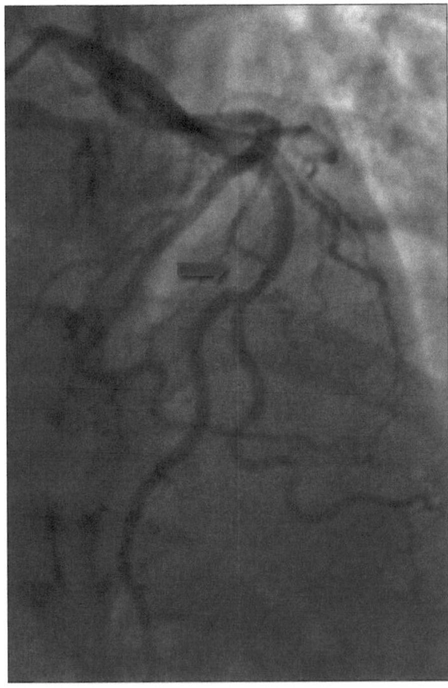

Figure 19: 37-year-old woman, hypertensive, previous MI. **Type 1 dissection of IVA III.**

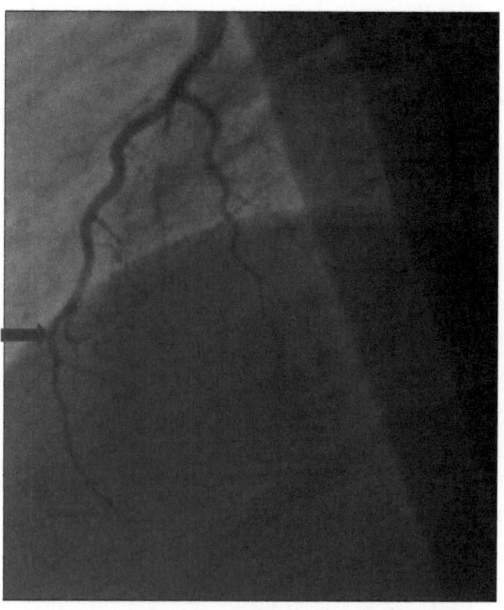

Figure 20: 35-year-old man, NSTEMI with normal ECG. **Type 2 dissection of IVA III** confirmed on MRI (transmural ischaemic contrast of the anterior wall).

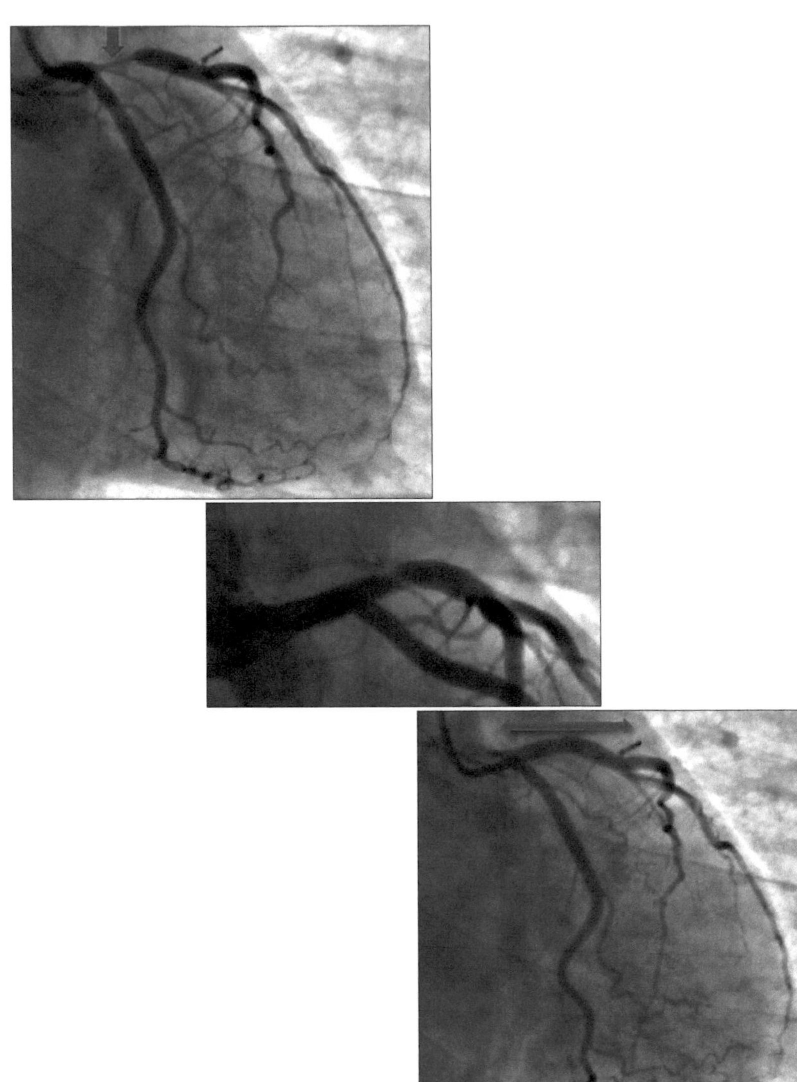

Figure 21: 63-year-old man, smoker, very high-risk NSTEMI. **Type 3 dissection of IVA I** (A). Extension of the dissection after angioplasty with an active stent (B). Final result after covering the dissection with a second active stent (C).

<u>Distal coronary involvement was therefore predominant in our series (10 patients, 77%)</u>.

IV - THERAPEUTIC MANAGEMENT :

Given the unstable presentation, all patients were initially put on double platelet anti-aggregation (Aspirin and Clopidogrel) with curative anticoagulation.

IV - 1 - Myocardial revascularisation :

Of the three patients with progressive MI, two underwent thrombolysis with failure (100%).

In our series, only three patients (23%) underwent percutaneous coronary intervention (PCI). Successful PCI was achieved in two patients (67%).

Conservative treatment was therefore the rule for the majority of patients (N=10, 77%) due to distal anatomical location or very extensive lesions (Table III).

No patient underwent coronary artery bypass grafting (CABG) following dissection.

Table III: Treatment modalities

	Clinical presentation	**Treatment**	**Receipt**	**Result if ICP**
Patient 1	Evolving IDM	*Thrombolysis* Treatment curator	-Distal seat (CD), TIMI 3	-
Patient 2	Evolving IDM	Curator	Extensive lesion (Mg), TIMI 3	-
Patient 3	Evolving IDM	*Thrombolysis* - PCI	Angina refractory, TIMI 1	Failure (Migration of the haematoma)
Patient 4	IDM seen late	Curator	Distal location (IVA), TIMI 3	-
Patient 5	MI seen late	ICP	Angina residual, IVA I, TIMI 0	Success
Patient 6	NSTEMI very high risk	ICP	IVA I, TIMI 2	Success

Patient 7	NSTEMI	Curator	Distal location (IVA), TIMI 3	-
Patient 8	NSTEMI	Curator	Distal location (IVA), TIMI 3	-
Patient 9	NSTEMI	Curator	Distal location (IVA), TIMI 3	-
Patient 10	NSTEMI	Curator	Distal location (IVA), TIMI 3	-
Patient 11	NSTEMI	Curator	Distal location (Mg), TIMI 3	-
Patient 12	NSTEMI	Curator	Length of CD lesion, TIMI 3	-
Patient 13	NSTEMI	Curator	Length of lesion Mg, TIMI 3	-

RCA: right coronary artery; PCI: percutaneous coronary intervention; MI: myocardial infarction; AVI: anterior interventricular; Mg: marginal; NSTEMI: non-ST-segment elevation myocardial infarction.

IV - 2 - Medical treatment on discharge :

Beta-blockers, aspirin and clopidogrel were prescribed for the majority of patients (12, 11 and 10 respectively) (Table IV).

Antihypertensive treatment with converting enzyme inhibitors (CEIs) or angiotensin II receptor antagonists (ARBs) was also prescribed in eight patients.

Acenocoumarol was started in the patient with an apical thrombus.

Table IV: Medical treatment at discharge

Treatment	Number of patients (%)
Aspirin	11 (85%)
Clopidogrel	10 (77%)
Beta-blocker	12 (92%)
IEC/ARA II	8 (61%)
Statin	9 (69%)
Calcium inhibitor	3 (23%)
Diuretic	1 (8%)
Anti-aldosterone	0 (0%)
Nitro derivative	3 (23%)
Acenocoumarol	1 (8%)

ACE inhibitor: ACE inhibitor; ARB II: angiotensin II receptor antagonist.

IV - IN-HOSPITAL AND LONG-TERM FOLLOW-UP :

IV - 1 - In-hospital monitoring

The median length of stay in hospital was 5 days, with extremes ranging from 4 to 17 days.

No MACCE was noted during the hospital stay.

It should be noted that one patient presented with haematemesis following thrombolysis with deglobulation, requiring transfusion and endoscopic treatment (placement of two clips on a deepening oesophageal ulcer) with a good subsequent outcome. The patient was discharged on clopidogrel to replace aspirin with gastric protection.

IV - 2 - Long-term monitoring

All patients were followed prospectively and none were lost to follow-up.

The median follow-up was 18 months, with extremes ranging from 0.6 to 25.3 months.

No MACCE was reported during follow-up.

No patient was readmitted to hospital or had an angiographic check-up. Mortality and the rate of MACCE at the end of this follow-up in our series was 0%.

Discussion

I - HISTOPATHOLOGY OF SPONTANEOUS CORONARY ARTERY DISSECTION

CASD results from the development of a haematoma in the tunica media leading to separation of the intima or intima-media complex from the underlying vessel, resulting in compression of the true lumen (11- 13).

The main cause of the formation of the false lumen is not well elucidated, with two hypotheses having been proposed to explain the pathophysiological process: the "Inside-out" model, where the causal event is the development of an endothelial and intimal tear, allowing blood to cross the internal elastic boundary and accumulate in the media, and the "Inside-out" model, where the causal event is the development of an endothelial and intimal tear, allowing blood to cross the internal elastic boundary and accumulate in the media.

"outside-in" (Figure 22) where the causal event is rupture of the vasa vasorum leading to haemorrhage directly into the media (14,15).

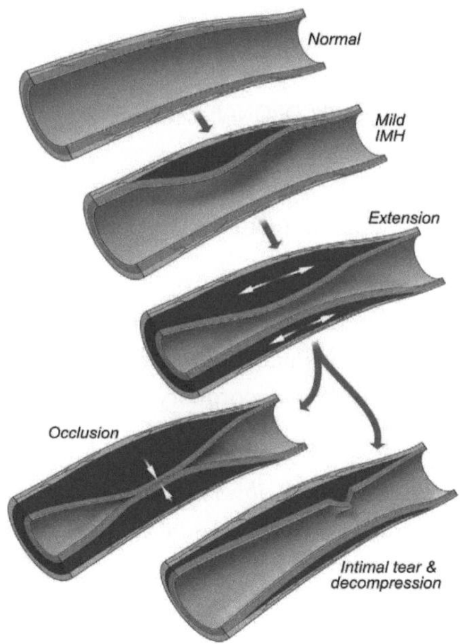

Figure 22: The "outside-in" mechanism of dissection, after Hayes et al (8).

In both cases, the blood spreads axially as the false channel expands, leading to compression of the true channel.

We still don't know whether there is a single mechanism in the CASDs or whether both mechanisms are possible.

Three phenomena favour the "outside-in" mechanism:

1) The majority of DSAC cases show no communication between the true and false channels (14,16,17).

2) Serial angiograms performed early after CASD indicate that intramural haematoma precedes the development of intimal dissection (14).

3) Recent imaging studies with optical coherence tomography (OCT) show that the false lumen is pressurised and that the fenestrations observed may result from the rupture of the false lumen into the true lumen rather than vice versa (17).

Although the majority of DSACs are probably due to an 'outside-in' mechanism, the phenotype of a given dissection could result from several pathophysiological sequences.

II - EPIDEMIOLOGY OF SPONTANEOUS CORONARY ARTERY DISSECTION

II - 1 - Impact

The true incidence of CASD remains unknown because the condition is under-diagnosed (18).

CASD was historically considered to be a very rare angiographic finding, but contemporary series report an incidence of CASD of 0.07 to 0.2% of all coronary angiographies and 2 to 4% of coronary angiographies performed for ACS (19-21).

These incidences are similar to those observed in our series, with 0.9% and 2.6% of all coronary angiographies and those performed in the context of ACS respectively.

II - 2 - Demographic characteristics

II - 2 - 1 - Age

Previously considered mainly a disease of young adults, CASD is now described in patients aged between 18 and 84 years (22,23), with the average age in large contemporary series ranging from 44 to 53 years (24-28).

In our series, the average age was 56.

II - 2 - 2 - Gender

The vast majority of DSAC patients (90%) are female (16,19,24,29).

The predilection of CASD for female patients and the association with pregnancy suggest a pathophysiological role for female sex hormones.

Male patients appear to differ from female cases, being slightly younger and with onset favoured by intense physical exercise rather than emotional stress (30).

In our series, and in line with the demographic data from international series, there was a marked predominance of women, with 85% of DSAC cases being female.

II - 2 - 3 - Cardiovascular risk factors :

Atherosclerosis is rare in the typical CASD.

Patients with CAD have fewer of the traditional cardiovascular risk factors of ischaemic heart disease than patients with atherosclerotic coronary artery disease (22), and some patients have no CVRF at all.

However, many patients have certain risk factors for ischaemic heart disease, including hypertension, smoking and dyslipidaemia (Table V), although there is no evidence that these contribute directly to the risk of CAD.

It should be noted that diabetes appears to be rare in patients with SCAD. Finally, as in the general population, FRCVs tend to be more frequent in older patients with SCAD.

In our series, only two patients (15%) had more than one FRCV.

Comparison of the demographic characteristics of our population with those of contemporary series (23-27,31,32) and with Saadi's national study (33) is summarised in Table V.

Table V: Demographic characteristics of the various contemporary series

	N patients	Age	Female(%)	HTA(%)	Chol(%)	Smoking(%)	Diabetes(%)
Mayo Clinic (2014) (24)	189	44 ± 9	92	31	22	15	2
Saw et al (2014) (23)	168	52 ± 9	92	39	24	13	5
Lettieri et al (2015) (25)	134	52 ± 11	81	51	33	34	2
Faden et al (2016) (26)	79	33 ± 5	100	17	18	17	11
Rogowski et al (2017) (27)	64	53 ± 11	94	45	52	28	0
Nakashima et al (2016) (31)	63	46 ± 10	94	33	23	32	0
Motreff et al (2017) (32)	55	50	100	27	11	22	4
Saadi (2018) (33)	43	45 ± 10	60	14	2	30	9
Our series (2020)	**13**	**56 ± 11**	**85**	**38**	**8**	**23**	**8**

II - 3 - Associated conditions

The pathophysiology of CASD remains unknown. It is likely that a combination of predisposing factors increase susceptibility so that a minor triggering event is sufficient to precipitate dissection.

Predispositions :

Fibromuscular dysplasia

Coronary tortuosities (9) **and coronary aneurysms Pregnancy (antepartum, postpartum, multiple pregnancies) Connective tissue diseases**

Marfan syndrome Loeys-Dietz syndrome

Ehler Danlos syndrome type IV Neurofibromatosis type I

Medial cystic necrosis Lysyl oxidase deficiency Alpha-1 antitrypsin deficiency Alport syndrome Polycystic kidney disease Pseudoxanthoma elasticum

Therapy / Hormonal imbalance

Menstruation (34) Post-abortion Oral contraception

Hormone replacement therapy Clomiphene

≥-HCG

Testosterone

Polycystic ovary syndrome

Systemic disease

Systemic lupus erythematosus

Inflammatory bowel disease Polyarteritis nodosa

Sarcoidosis

Churg-Strauss syndrome Wegener's syndrome Rheumatoid arthritis (23) Takayasu syndrome (35) Hypothyroidism (36)

Celiac disease (37) Vaquez's disease (38) Behcet's disease (39) Cryoglobulinemia

Precipitating factors:

Coronary spasm (40,41)

Intense exercise (isometric, aerobic)

Emotional stress (23,30,31)

Recreational drugs Cocaine Amphetamines

Sleep deprivation (42)

Valsalva-type activities (sexual activity (43), vomiting (44), coughing (45), etc.) **Medications**: Calcineurin inhibitors (ciclosporin, tacrolimus, vaclosporin), 5-FU (46), fenfluramine, corticosteroids (47), methylphenidate, ergotamine, sumatriptan, hepersensitivity reactions (48), dobutamine (49).

II - 3 - 1- Pregnancy

Pregnancy and peripartum cases represent a minority of DSACs (around 10% in most contemporary series).

As a result, CASD should no longer be considered primarily as a peripartum condition.

However, 21-27% of myocardial infarctions during pregnancy and 50% of post-partum coronary events are thought to be due to CASD.

The precise nature of this association remains to be elucidated, but it may be linked to hormonal influences on vascular connective tissue and/or vascular micro-vascularisation.

In our series, there were no cases of CASD associated with pregnancy.

II - 3 - 2- Fibromuscular dysplasia

CASD has been associated with various predisposing arteriopathies. The most common is fibromuscular dysplasia (FMD).

FMD is a non-atherosclerotic, non-inflammatory disease of the arterial walls, which also occurs mainly in middle-aged women with few risk factors.

It can lead to stenoses, dissections and aneurysms of medium-sized arteries, including but not limited to renal, cervicocephalic and visceral arteries.

Although FMD is the most common extracoronary vascular anomaly in patients with CAD, patients without imaging evidence of FMD were reported to have other arterial anomalies, including coronary or extracoronary dissections, aneurysms or tortuosity (78%).

Some of these patients may have typical MFD that has not been identified due to incomplete or insufficiently sensitive imaging techniques.

Also, no therapeutic intervention was described by the authors who diagnosed asymptomatic extra-coronary FMD.

In our series, no cases of FMD have been reported.

II - 3 - 3- Systemic inflammatory diseases

CASD has been associated with systemic inflammatory diseases.

While the prevalence of this association was 8.9% in the series by Saw et al (23), this data has not been widely corroborated in other series (16). A clear link between systemic inflammation and CASD remains to be elucidated.

In our series, two women had hypothyroidism on replacement therapy, an association reported by Ionescu et al (36) in 2009.

III - CLINICAL PRESENTATIONS

There is clear evidence that SCAD remains under-diagnosed (18). Some patients do not pay attention to their symptoms and never go to emergency, while others may present with sudden death straight away.

However, for those who do consult, a missed or delayed DSAC diagnosis is common (6.50).

Some patients are not referred for coronary angiography, mainly because most medical and cardiology services are focused on identifying patients at high ischaemic risk, whereas patients with SCAD generally fall into the lowest risk group on the basis of traditional risk scores for ischaemic heart disease. A high suspicion of CASD in typical patients, coupled with knowledge of the angiographic variants of CASD is essential to minimise missed or delayed diagnoses.

CASD patients generally present with ACS associated with positive myocardial necrosis biomarkers.

The proportion of cases presenting STEMI (26 to 55%) compared with NSTEMI varies according to the series, probably reflecting differences in selection for these registries.

In our series, five patients (39%) presented with STEMI. Of these, two (40%) were seen late.

IV - ANGIOGRAPHIC DIAGNOSIS

Differential diagnoses of CASD include atherosclerotic ACS, coronary spasm, Takotsubo cardiomyopathy, embolic infarction and myocardial infarction with non-obstruction of the coronary arteries (MINOCA).

There is currently no blood biomarker for the diagnosis of CAD. Coronary angiography is the main diagnostic tool in clinical practice.

Intracoronary injection of nitrates is mandatory when invasive pressure allows, to ensure complete vasodilatation and exclude the possibility of associated coronary spasm.

With experience, most cases of CASD can be diagnosed on angiography alone, with endo-coronary imaging reserved for cases of diagnostic uncertainty (6).

However, it is important to note that aspects of intimal flap, double lumen and parietal stagnation of contrast medium, classic images seen with iatrogenic dissections (51) and familiar to most interventional cardiologists, are only present in a minority of angiograms of DSACs.

According to the classification by Saw et al (3), type 2 is the most frequent, followed by type 1 (23,27,31). Types 3 and 4 are the least frequent.

Other angiographic features reported in association with CASD :

- An increase in coronary tortuosity (9)
- Predilection for more distal coronary segments (in contrast to atherosclerosis) (23,25,27)
- predominant involvement of the IVA and its branches (23,25,31,32)
- A false lumen starting and/or ending at a collateral branch (32)
- Absence or reduced incidence of co-existing atherosclerosis, with unaffected coronaries generally normal or almost normal (32)
- The DFM
- The association of dissection sites with intramyocardial tracts (52)

In our series, and in accordance with the data in the literature, we note :

- *Predominance of type 2 (46%), with types 1 and 2 accounting for 84% of diagnosed CASDs*
- *Coronary tortuosities present in 38% of cases*
- *Distal arterial involvement in 77% of cases*
- *Most of the damage was to the VIA (54%)*

Endo-coronary imaging was not used in our series due to a lack of availability in our catheterisation laboratory.

Cardiac MRI was useful on two occasions in establishing a diagnosis of acute ischaemic damage (characterised by transmural uptake of

gadolinium) in the presence of a normal coronary appearance and a strong suspicion of DSAC.

The advantages of endo-coronary imaging for the diagnosis of CAD :

- Final diagnosis from DSAC
- Confirms the position of the coronary guide in the true channel in the case of PCI
- Facilitates stent sizing
- Confirms correct stent placement
- Confirms complete coverage of the dissected segment
- Facilitates diagnosis of probable associated arterial disease

The disadvantages of endo-coronary imaging in CASD :

- Invasive method, requiring anticoagulation
- Limited availability
- Risk of extension of the dissection by :
- guide catheter or coronary guide
- the imaging catheter
- hydraulic extension with OCT
- Risk of vascular occlusion (by catheter, embolisation)

Overall, while the diagnosis at coronary angiography remains uncertain, the 2018 US recommendations (5) **suggest:**

- **Use of OCT or IVUS if feasible and without risk**
- **Coroscan (especially if proximal lesion)**
- **The search for extracoronary vascular anomalies (ECV)**
- **Repeat the coronary angiography after 6 to 8 weeks.**

IV - TREATMENT :

IV - 1 - Thrombolysis :

Although individual historical cases of DSAC apparently being successfully thrombolysed have been described, extensions of dissection and even coronary ruptures leading to tamponade after lytic treatment have been reported.

Thrombolysis is therefore contraindicated for the acute management of CASD.

In our series, two STEMIs were thrombolysed without success.

IV - 2 - Conservative treatment, PCI or CABG?

IV - 2 - 1 - Conservative treatment

There is strong evidence that the majority of DSACs will initially stabilise and then heal completely over time if managed conservatively (16,23,24,27,31).

Revascularisation in patients with CAD is very difficult due to the presence of a disrupted and friable underlying coronary vessel wall. This explains the poorer results of PCI in SCAD compared with atherosclerotic stenosis (24,25,27,31).

For this reason, a conservative strategy should be favoured whenever revascularisation is not mandatory (i.e. in haemodynamically stable patients without progressive ischaemia and with normal flow in the culprit artery) (6,18).

In our series, conservative treatment was used in the majority of cases (77%).

IV - 2 - 2 - Percutaneous coronary intervention

Published studies show an increased risk of PCI complications during DSAC.

In the Canadian series by Saw et al (23), procedural success was achieved in only 64% of patients.

In the large Mayo Clinic series (Tweet et al.) (24), procedural success was achieved in only 57% of cases.

Furthermore, revascularisation was not associated with a reduced long-term risk of repeat revascularisation or recurrent DSAC.

In the event of ischaemia or progressive infarction requiring intervention, interventional cardiologists need to be aware of the specific additional risks associated with interventions in DSACs. These include:

- Increased risk of secondary iatrogenic dissection
- Passage of the coronary guide through the false channel
- Proximal or distal propagation of IMH during stent deployment
- Persistent distal dissection
- Occlusion of the major collateral branches by propagation of the haematoma

Given the increased risk of angioplasty failure in CASD, a number of less conventional interventional approaches have been reported.

These include :

- Minimal balloon angioplasty to restore flow followed by a conservative strategy (53)
- Extended stent lengths to reduce the risk of haematoma spread
- Cover the proximal and distal ends of the affected segments with short stents to limit haematoma before stenting the intermediate segment (54,55).
- Targeting the intimal tear with a focal stent (31,56)
- Cutting balloon to fenestrate the intima-media membrane and decompress the false lumen as a stand-alone strategy possibly followed by stenting (57-60).

In our series, three PCIs were performed in the context of DSAC, with a success rate of 67% comparable to that reported in the literature.

There was one failure due to arterial occlusion caused by distal migration of the haematoma, and one complication of PCI, namely a persistent distal dissection successfully managed by a second stent.

IV - 2 - 3 - Aorto-coronary bypass surgery

CABG in DSAC is generally used as a bail-out strategy following failed angioplasty with progressive ischaemia or because the site and extent of the dissection (usually involving the TCG or the presence of multiple dissections) is felt to pose a prohibitive risk with conservative treatment or PCI.

Successful CABG can be difficult when dissection extends beyond the graft anastomosis site and great care must be taken to perform the anastomosis in the true lumen.

The literature on CAP in CASD is limited to small case series (5 to 23 cases).

High rates of graft failure have been reported, possibly due to healing of the native network leading to competitive flow and secondary graft thrombosis (24).

In our series, there were no cases of CAP during a DSAC.

IV - 3 - Medical treatment

To date, there are no randomised controlled trials comparing different pharmacological treatment strategies for CASD.

Current practice is therefore based on observations of cases and registers and the extrapolation (where possible) of guidelines for the treatment of ACS not linked to a CASD.

IV - 3 - 1 - Anticoagulant treatment

Anticoagulation should be limited to acute administration during revascularisation procedures, while chronic use should be restricted to situations where there is an unequivocal clinical indication (such as left ventricular thrombus or thromboembolic events) (6).

In our series, only one patient was kept on anticoagulant treatment due to the presence of an apical thrombus on TTE.

IV - 3 - 2 - Antithrombotic treatments

The use of antiplatelet agents and the duration of treatment remains an area of controversy with divergent practices within SCAD. This stems from an apparent conflict between existing evidence of efficacy in non-CAD ACS versus an inherent (albeit unproven) concern about the use of these drugs prolonging bleeding time in a disease whose primary pathophysiology may be intramural haemorrhage (6).

This can be further complicated by problematic menorrhagia which can be a problem in survivors of CAD of childbearing age taking antiplatelet agents (61).

Patients who undergo stenting should receive double platelet anti-aggregation for 12 months and prolonged or lifelong monotherapy (usually with aspirin) in accordance with ACS recommendations. In conservatively treated patients, there is evidence from OCT studies of significant stenosis sometimes associated with thrombus in DSACs (2).

This justifies antiplatelet therapy in the acute phase and most authors recommend dual antiplatelet therapy in the acute phase (generally with aspirin and clopidogrel rather than the new P2Y12 inhibitors and avoiding intravenous antiaggregants) (62-64).

The optimal duration of subsequent monotherapy remains unknown, with some authors advocating long-term aspirin therapy (62,63) and others questioning this approach (64).

IV - 3 - 3 - ACE inhibitors, ARB II, beta-blockers, anti-aldosterone and nitrate derivatives

The medical management of patients with significantly impaired left ventricular function should follow heart failure guidelines and aim to titrate doses of ACE inhibitor or ARB II and beta-blockers, with a mineralocorticoid receptor antagonist added second, although hypotension frequently limits dose increases in this young population.

The management of CASD survivors without left ventricular dysfunction is more controversial. Beta-blocker treatment appears to reduce the risk of recurrence (63).

Vasodilators (e.g. nitrates or calcium channel blockers) are reserved for the empirical treatment of chest pain during the acute phase and following the index event.

IV - 3 - 4 - Statins

The justification for prescribing statins for a condition whose pathophysiology has no known association with cholesterol has not been established.

In general, statins are reserved for patients with a conventional indication for this treatment.

V - PROGNOSIS OF SPONTANEOUS CORONARY ARTERY DISSECTIONS :

In patients surviving DSAC, long-term mortality is low. In the American Mayo Clinic series (22), 10-year survival estimated by the Kaplan Meier curve was 92%.

A comparison of in-hospital and long-term mortality between the different series is summarised in Table VI.

Table VI: In-hospital and long-term mortality in the different series

Mortality hospital (%)		**Median follow-up (months)**	**Mortality at term of follow-up (%)**
Tweet et al (24)	0,5	27	1,6
Lettieri et al (25)	2,2	22	3,1
Rogowski et al (27)	2	54	0
Nakashima et al (31)	0	34	1,6
Saw et al (63)	0	37	1,2
Saadi (33)	6,9	36	5
Our series	0	18	0

VI - LIMITATIONS OF THE STUDY

- The small size of the study
- Monocentricity
- The absence of a comparison group with atherosclerosis-related ACS
- Lack of longer-term follow-up of patients to detect MACCE.
- Lack of availability of endo-coronary imaging techniques
- The absence of DFM screening
- Lack of angiographic control to confirm anatomical healing

CONCLUSIONS

CASD is a major cause of ACS in young and middle-aged people, particularly women without traditional cardiovascular risk factors.

It is frequently under-diagnosed or misdiagnosed and can potentially lead to significant morbidity and mortality.

Careful suspicion by the DSAC is necessary for diagnosis and treatment.

Despite growing recognition of this condition by both the medical community and patients, there are still major gaps in knowledge that need to be filled if the best results are to be achieved.

It must be acknowledged that most of the available data is retrospective and observational, and that the limited prospective studies are all recent.

Our work was a prospective monocentric study conducted in the cardiology department of Mongi Slim La Marsa Hospital over a two-year period from August 2018 to August 2020 and including 13 patients with DSAC.

The incidence of CASD in our study was 0.9% of all coronary angiographies and 2.6% of coronary angiographies performed for ACS.

The mean age was 56 ± 11 years, with a sex ratio of 0.2. The majority of patients (46%) had no FRCV.

No case of DSAC was related to pregnancy in our series. It should be noted that two patients had hypothyroidism under treatment.

The predominant clinical presentation was NSTEMI in 61% of cases (8 patients). Of these, only one was at very high risk.

Five patients (39%) had STEMI, three were progressive and two were seen on day 2.

Angiographically, type 2 was predominant (46%), with types 1 and 2 accounting for 84% of DSACs diagnosed, with the majority of cases involving the IVA (54%) and distal arteries in 77% of cases. Coronary tortuosities were associated in 38% of cases.

In terms of treatment, of the three patients with progressive MI, two underwent thrombolysis with failure (100%).

Only three patients (23%) underwent PCI. Successful PCI was achieved in two patients (67%).

Conservative treatment was therefore the rule for the majority of patients (10, 77%).

No patient had a CABG after dissection.

In-hospital mortality and mortality after a median follow-up of 18 months was 0%. Similarly, no MACCE was noted during the same follow-up period.

These results are in perfect agreement with the data in the contemporary literature, particularly concerning the incidence of SCAD, a clear predominance of women and an age of onset around fifty. Also, angiographically, there is preferential distal involvement of the AVI.

Thrombolysis is ineffective in this setting, and PCI is less likely to be successful.

Conservative treatment, still debated, remains the first-line treatment for these particular forms of MI.

REFERENCES

1. Pretty HC. Dissecting aneurysm of coronary artery in a woman aged 42: rupture. BMJ. 1931;(1):667.

2. Alfonso F, Paulo M, Gonzalo N, Dutary J, Jimenez-Quevedo P, Lennie V, et al. Diagnosis of Spontaneous Coronary Artery Dissection by Optical Coherence Tomography. Journal of the American College of Cardiology. March 2012;59(12):1073-9.

3. Saw J. Coronary angiogram classification of spontaneous coronary artery dissection: Coronary Angiogram Classification of Spontaneous Coronary Artery Dissection. Cathet Cardiovasc Intervent. 1 Dec 2014;84(7):1115-22.

4. Adlam D, Alfonso F, Maas A, Vrints C, Writing Committee, al-Hussaini A, et al. European Society of Cardiology, acute cardiovascular care association, SCAD study group: a position paper on spontaneous coronary artery dissection. European Heart Journal. 21 Sep 2018;39(36):3353-68.

5. Hayes SN, Kim ESH, Saw J, Adlam D, Arslanian-Engoren C, Economy KE, et al. Spontaneous Coronary Artery Dissection: Current State of the Science: A Scientific Statement From the American Heart Association. Circulation [Internet]. May 8, 2018;137(19).

6. Al-Hussaini A, Adlam D. Spontaneous coronary artery dissection. Heart. jul 2017;103(13):1043-51.

7. Huber MS, Mooney JF, Madison J, Mooney MR. Use of a morphologic classification to predict clinical outcome after dissection from coronary angioplasty. The American Journal of Cardiology. August 1991;68(5):467-71.

8. Hayes SN, Tweet MS, Adlam D, Kim ESH, Gulati R, Price JE, et al. Spontaneous Coronary Artery Dissection. Journal of the American College of Cardiology. August 2020;76(8):961-84.

9. Eleid MF, Guddeti RR, Tweet MS, Lerman A, Singh M, Best PJ, et al. Coronary Artery Tortuosity in Spontaneous Coronary Artery Dissection: Angiographic Characteristics and Clinical Implications. Circ Cardiovasc Interv. Oct 2014;7(5):656-62.

10. Cutlip DE, Windecker S, Mehran R, Boam A, Cohen DJ, van Es G-A, et al. Clinical end points in coronary stent trials: a case for standardized definitions. Circulation. 1 May 2007;115(17):2344-51.

11. R M, Eg B, Rf C. Eosinophilic Coronary Periarteritis with Arterial

Dissection: The Mast Cell Hypothesis. J Forensic Sci. March 16, 2015;60(4):1088-92.

12. Melez İ, Arslan M, Melez D, Akçay A, Büyük Y, Avşar A, et al. Spontaneous Coronary Artery Dissection: Report of 3 Cases and Literature Review Hormonal, Autoimmune, Morphological Factors. Am J Forensic Med Pathol. 1 Sep 2015;36(3):188-92.

13. Desai S, Sheppard MN. Sudden cardiac death: look closely at the coronaries for spontaneous dissection which can be missed. A study of 9 cases. Am J Forensic Med Pathol. March 2012;33(1):26-9.

14. Waterbury Thomas M., Tweet Marysia S., Hayes Sharonne N., Eleid Mackram F., Bell Malcolm R., Lerman Amir, et al. Early Natural History of Spontaneous Coronary Artery Dissection. Circulation: Cardiovascular Interventions. Sep 1, 2018;11(9):e006772.

15. Waterbury TM, Tarantini G, Vogel B, Mehran R, Gersh BJ, Gulati R. Non-atherosclerotic causes of acute coronary syndromes. Nature Reviews Cardiology. Apr 2020;17(4):229-41.

16. Alfonso F, Paulo M, Lennie V, Dutary J, Bernardo E, Jiménez-Quevedo P, et al. Spontaneous Coronary Artery Dissection: Long-Term Follow-Up of a Large Series of Patients Prospectively Managed With a "Conservative" Therapeutic Strategy. JACC: Cardiovascular Interventions. 1 Oct 2012;5(10):1062-70.

17. Jackson R, Al-Hussaini A, Joseph S, van Soest G, Wood A, Macaya F, et al. Spontaneous Coronary Artery Dissection: Pathophysiological Insights From Optical Coherence Tomography. JACC: Cardiovascular Imaging. Dec 1, 2019;12(12):2475-88.

18. Tweet MS, Gulati R, Hayes SN. Spontaneous coronary artery dissection. Curr Cardiol Rep. 2016;18(7):60.

19. Vanzetto G, Berger-Coz E, Barone-Rochette G, Chavanon O, Bouvaist H, Hacini R, et al. Prevalence, therapeutic management and medium-term prognosis of spontaneous coronary artery dissection: results from a database of 11,605 patients. Eur J Cardiothorac Surg. Feb 2009;35(2):250-4.

20. Nishiguchi T, Tanaka A, Ozaki Y, Taruya A, Fukuda S, Taguchi H, et al. Prevalence of spontaneous coronary artery dissection in patients with acute

coronary syndrome. European Heart Journal: Acute Cardiovascular Care. June 2016;5(3):263-70.

21. Mortensen KH, Thuesen L, Kristensen IB, Christiansen EH. Spontaneous coronary artery dissection: a Western Denmark Heart Registry study. Catheter Cardiovasc Interv. 1 Nov 2009;74(5):710-7.

22. Tweet MS, Hayes SN, Pitta SR, Simari RD, Lerman A, Lennon RJ, et al. Clinical features, management, and prognosis of spontaneous coronary artery dissection. Circulation. 31 Jul 2012;126(5):579-88.

23. Saw J, Aymong E, Sedlak T, Buller CE, Starovoytov A, Ricci D, et al. Spontaneous coronary artery dissection: association with predisposing arteriopathies and precipitating stressors and cardiovascular outcomes. Circ Cardiovasc Interv. Oct 2014;7(5):645-55.

24. Tweet MS, Eleid MF, Best PJM, Lennon RJ, Lerman A, Rihal CS, et al. Spontaneous coronary artery dissection: revascularization versus conservative therapy. Circ Cardiovasc Interv. Dec 2014;7(6):777-86.

25. Lettieri C, Zavalloni D, Rossini R, Morici N, Ettori F, Leonzi O, et al. Management and Long-Term Prognosis of Spontaneous Coronary Artery Dissection. Am J Cardiol. 1 Jul 2015;116(1):66-73.

26. Faden MS, Bottega N, Benjamin A, Brown RN. A nationwide evaluation of spontaneous coronary artery dissection in pregnancy and the puerperium. Heart. 15 2016;102(24):1974-9.

27. Rogowski S, Maeder MT, Weilenmann D, Haager PK, Ammann P, Rohner F, et al. Spontaneous Coronary Artery Dissection: Angiographic Follow-Up and Long-Term Clinical Outcome in a Predominantly Medically Treated Population. Catheter Cardiovasc Interv. Jan 2017;89(1):59-68.

28. Rashid HNZ, Wong DTL, Wijesekera H, Gutman SJ, Shanmugam VB, Gulati R, et al. Incidence and characterisation of spontaneous coronary artery dissection as a cause of acute coronary syndrome--A single-centre Australian experience. Int J Cardiol. 1 Jan 2016;202:336-8.

29. Elkayam U, Jalnapurkar S, Barakkat MN, Khatri N, Kealey AJ, Mehra A, et al. Pregnancy-associated acute myocardial infarction: a review of contemporary experience in 150 cases between 2006 and 2011. Circulation. 22 Apr 2014;129(16):1695-702.

30. Fahmy P, Prakash R, Starovoytov A, Boone R, Saw J. Pre-Disposing and

Precipitating Factors in Men With Spontaneous Coronary Artery Dissection. JACC Cardiovasc Interv. Apr 25, 2016;9(8):866-8.

31. Nakashima T, Noguchi T, Haruta S, Yamamoto Y, Oshima S, Nakao K, et al. Prognostic impact of spontaneous coronary artery dissection in young female patients with acute myocardial infarction: A report from the Angina Pectoris-Myocardial Infarction Multicenter Investigators in Japan. Int J Cardiol. 15 March 2016;207:341-8.

32. Motreff P, Malcles G, Combaret N, Barber-Chamoux N, Bouajila S, Pereira B, et al. How and when to suspect spontaneous coronary artery dissection: novel insights from a single-centre series on prevalence and angiographic appearance. EuroIntervention. 7 Apr 2017;12(18):e2236-43.

33. Saadi, Mohamed. Management and long-term prognosis of spontaneous coronary artery dissection: a national multicenter study. Tunis Faculty of Medicine; 2018.

34. Marcoff, Rahman. Menstruation-associated spontaneous coronary artery dissection. J Invasive Cardiol. 1 Oct 2010;22(10):E183-5.

35. Gerede DM, Yüksel B, Tutar E, Küçükşahin O, Uzun C, Atasoy KÇ, et al. Spontaneous Coronary Artery Dissection in a Male Patient with Takayasu's Arteritis and Antiphospholipid Antibody Syndrome. Case Rep Rheumatol. 2013;2013:272963.

36. Ionescu C, Chrissoheris M, Caraccciolo E. Spontaneous coronary artery dissection and severe hypothyroidism [Internet]. Vol. 21, The Journal of invasive cardiology. J Invasive Cardiol; 2009 [cited 12 Sep 2020]. Available from: https://pubmed.ncbi.nlm.nih.gov/19342762/

37. Bayar N, Çağırcı G, Üreyen ÇM, Kuş G, Küçükseymen S, Arslan Ş. The Relationship between Spontaneous Multi-Vessel Coronary Artery Dissection and Celiac Disease. Korean Circ J. May 2015;45(3):242-4.

38. Kay IP, Williams MJ. Spontaneous coronary artery dissection: long stenting in a patient with polycythemia vera. Int J Cardiovasc Intervent. 1999;2(3):191-3.

39. Buccheri D, Piraino D, Andolina G. Behçet disease and spontaneous coronary artery dissection: The chicken or the egg? Int J Cardiol. 19 Apr 2016;215:504-5.

40. Tsujita K, Miyazaki T, Kaikita K, Chitose T, Takaoka N, Soejima H, et al.

Premenopausal woman with acute myocardial infarction caused by spontaneous coronary artery dissection and potential association with coronary vasospasm. Cardiovasc Interv Ther. 7 Feb 2012;27(2):121-6.

41. Reriani M, Sara J, Flammer A, Gulati R, Li J, Rihal C, et al. Coronary endothelial function testing provides superior discrimination compared with standard clinical risk scoring in prediction of cardiovascular events. Coron Artery Dis. May 1, 2016;27(3):213-20.

42. Suh SY, Kim JW, Choi CU, Kim EJ, Rha S-W, Park CG, et al. Spontaneous coronary dissection associated with sleep deprivation presenting with acute myocardial infarction. Int J Cardiol. Feb 7, 2007;115(2):e78-79.

43. Schifferdecker B, Pacifico L, Ramsaran EK, Folland ED, Spodick DH, Weiner BH. Spontaneous coronary artery dissection associated with sexual intercourse. Am J Cardiol. May 15, 2004;93(10):1323-4.

44. Velusamy M, Fisherkeller M, Keenan M, Kiernan F, Fram D. Spontaneous coronary artery dissection in a young woman precipitated by retching. J Invasive Cardiol. 1 Apr 2002;14(4):198-201.

45. Sivam S, Yozghatlian V, Dentice R, McGrady M, Moriarty C, Di Michiel J, et al. Spontaneous coronary artery dissection associated with coughing. Journal of Cystic Fibrosis. march 2014;13(2):235-7.

46. Hart K, Patel S, Kovoor J. Spontaneous Coronary Artery Dissection Associated with Anal Cancer Management with Fluorouracil and Radiotherapy. Cureus [Internet]. [cited 2020 Sep 12];11(6). Available from: https://www.ncbi.nlm.nih.gov/pmc/articles/PMC6706264/

47. Keir ML, Dehghani P. Corticosteroids and Spontaneous Coronary Artery Dissection: A New Predisposing Factor? Can J Cardiol. March 2016;32(3):395.e7-8.

48. Saunders SL, Ford SE. Primary coronary artery dissection possibly related to drug hypersensitivity in a male. Can J Cardiol. Apr 1991;7(3):138-40.

49. Karabinos I, Papadopoulos A, Koulouris S, Kranidis A, Korovesis S, Katritsis D. Spontaneous coronary artery dissection during a dobutamine stress echocardiography. Echocardiography. March 2006;23(3):232-4.

50. Saw J, Humphries K, Aymong E, Sedlak T, Prakash R, Starovoytov A, et al. Spontaneous coronary artery dissection. Journal of the American

College of Cardiology. august 2017;70(9):1148-58.

51. Rogers JH, Lasala JM. Coronary artery dissection and perforation complicating percutaneous coronary intervention. J Invasive Cardiol. Sept 2004;16(9):493-9.

52. De-Giorgio F, Grassi VM, Abbate A, d'Aloja E, Arena V. Causation or coincidence? A case of sudden death due to spontaneous coronary artery dissection in presence of myocardial bridging. Int J Cardiol. 23 August 2012;159(2):e32-34.

53. Arrivi A, Milici C, Bock C, Placanica A, Boschetti E, Dominici M. Idiopathic, Serial Coronary Vessels Dissection in a Young Woman with Psychological Stress: A Case Report and Review of the Literature. Case Rep Vasc Med [Internet]. 2012 [cited 2020 Sep 12];2012. Available from: https://www.ncbi.nlm.nih.gov/pmc/articles/PMC3485898/

54. Walsh SJ, Jokhi PP, Saw J. Successful percutaneous management of coronary dissection and extensive intramural haematoma associated with ST elevation MI. Acute Card Care. 2008;10(4):231-3.

55. Dashwood AM, Saw J, Dhillon P, Murdoch D. Use of a Three-Stent Technique for a Case of Spontaneous Coronary Artery Dissection. Can J Cardiol. 2017;33(6):830.e13-830.e15.

56. Alfonso F, Bastante T, García-Guimaraes M, Pozo E, Cuesta J, Rivero F, et al. Spontaneous coronary artery dissection: new insights into diagnosis and treatment. Coron Artery Dis. Dec 2016;27(8):696-706.

57. Ito T, Shintani Y, Ichihashi T, Fujita H, Ohte N. Non-atherosclerotic spontaneous coronary artery dissection revascularized by intravascular ultrasonography-guided fenestration with cutting balloon angioplasty. Cardiovasc Interv Ther. Jul 2017;32(3):241-3.

58. Alkhouli M, Cole M, Ling FS. Coronary artery fenestration prior to stenting in spontaneous coronary artery dissection. Catheter Cardiovasc Interv. Jul 2016;88(1):E23-27.

59. Motreff P, Barber-Chamoux N, Combaret N, Souteyrand G. Coronary artery fenestration guided by optical coherence tomography before stenting: new interventional option in rescue management of compressive spontaneous intramural hematoma. Circ Cardiovasc Interv. Apr 2015;8(4):e002266.

60. Yumoto K, Sasaki H, Aoki H, Kato K. Successful treatment of spontaneous coronary artery dissection with cutting balloon angioplasty as evaluated with optical coherence tomography. JACC Cardiovasc Interv. Jul 2014;7(7):817-9.

61. Maas AHEM, Euler M von, Bongers MY, Rolden HJA, Grutters JPC, Ulrich L, et al. Practice points in gynecardiology: Abnormal uterine bleeding in premenopausal women taking oral anticoagulant or antiplatelet therapy. Maturitas. dec 2015;82(4):355-9.

62. Saw J, Ricci D, Starovoytov A, Fox R, Buller CE. Spontaneous coronary artery dissection: prevalence of predisposing conditions including fibromuscular dysplasia in a tertiary center cohort. JACC Cardiovasc Interv. Jan 2013;6(1):44-52.

63. Saw J, Humphries K, Aymong E, Sedlak T, Prakash R, Starovoytov A, et al. Spontaneous Coronary Artery Dissection: Clinical Outcomes and Risk of Recurrence. J Am Coll Cardiol. August 29, 2017;70(9):1148-58.

64. Liang JJ, Prasad M, Tweet MS, Hayes SN, Gulati R, Breen JF, et al. A novel application of CT angiography to detect extracoronary vascular abnormalities in patients with spontaneous coronary artery dissection. J Cardiovasc Comput Tomogr. June 2014;8(3):189-97.

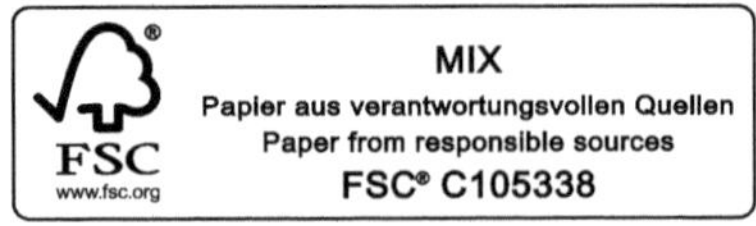

Printed by Books on Demand GmbH, Norderstedt / Germany